Hypochondriasis / A Practical Treatise (1766)

John Hill

INTRODUCTION

"When I first dabbled in this art, the old distemper call'd *Melancholy* was exchang'd for *Vapours*, and afterwards for the *Hypp*, and at last took up the now current appellation of the *Spleen*, which it still retains, tho' a learned doctor of the west, in a little tract he hath written, divides the *Spleen* and *Vapours*, not only into the *Hypp*, the *Hyppos*, and the Hyppocons; but subdivides these divisions into the *Markambles*, the *Moonpalls*, the *Strong-Fiacs*, and the *Hockogrokles*."

Nicholas Robinson, *A New System of the Spleen, Vapours, and Hypochondriack Melancholy* (London, 1729)

Treatises on hypochondriasis—the seventeenth-century medical term for a wide range of nervous diseases—were old when "Sir" John Hill, the eccentric English scientist, physician, apothecary, and hack writer, published his *Hypochondriasis* in 1766.[1] For at least a century and a half medical writers as well as lay authors had been writing literature of all types (treatises, pamphlets, poems, sermons, epigrams) on this most fashionable of English maladies under the variant names of "melancholy," "the spleen," "black melancholy," "hysteria," "nervous debility," "the hyp." Despite the plethora of *materia scripta* on the subject it makes sense to reprint Hill's *Hypochondriasis*, because it is indeed a "practical treatise" and because it offers the modern student of neoclassical literature a clear summary of the best thoughts that had been put forth on the subject, as well as an explanation of the causes, symptoms, and cures of this commonplace malady.

No reader of seventeenth- and eighteenth-century English literature needs to be reminded of the interest of writers of the period in the condition—"disease" is too confining a term—hypochondriasis.[2] Their concern is apparent in both the poetry and prose of two centuries. From Robert Burton's Brobdingnagian exposition in *The Anatomy of Melancholy* (1621) to Tobias Smollett's depiction of the misanthropic and ailing Matthew Bramble in *Humphry Clinker* (1771), and, of course, well into the nineteenth century, afflicted heroes and weeping heroines populate the pages of England's literature. There is scarcely a decade in the period 1600-1800 that does not contribute to the literature of melancholy; so considerable in number are the works that could be placed under this heading that it actually makes sense to speak of the "literature of melancholy." A kaleidoscopic survey of this literature (exclusive of treatises written on the subject) would include mention of Milton's "Il Penseroso" and "L'Allegro," the meditative Puritan and nervous Anglican thinkers of the Restoration (many of whose narrators, such as Richard Baxter, author of the *Reliquiae Baxterianae*,[3] are afflicted), Swift's "School of Spleen" in *A Tale of a Tub*, Pope's hysterical Belinda in the "Cave of Spleen," the melancholic "I" of Samuel Richardson's correspondence, Gray's leucocholy, the psychosomatically ailing characters of *The Vicar of Wakefield* and *Tristram Shandy*, Boswell's *Hypochondriack Papers* (1777-1783) contributed to the *London Magazine*, and such "sensible" and "sensitive" women as Mrs. Bennett and Miss Bates in the novels of Jane Austen. So great in bulk is this literature in the mid eighteenth century, that C. A. Moore has written, "statistically, this deserves to be called the Age of Melancholy."[4] The vastness of this literature is sufficient to justify the reprinting of an unavailable practical handbook on the subject by a prolific author all too little known.[5]

  The medical background of Hill's pamphlet extends further back than the seventeenth century and Burton's *Anatomy*. The ancient Greeks had theorized about hypochondria: ὑποχόνδριασις signified a disorder beneath (ὑπό) the gristle (χόνδρια) and the disease was discussed principally in physiological terms. The belief that hypochondriasis was a somatic condition persisted until the second half of the seventeenth century at which time an innovation was made by Dr. Thomas Sydenham. In addition to showing that hypochondriasis and hysteria (thought previously by Sydenham to afflict women only) were the same disease, Sydenham noted that the external cause of both was a mental disturbance and not a physiological one. He also had a theory that the internal and immediate cause was a disorder of the animal spirits arising from a clot and resulting in pain, spasms, and bodily disorders. By attributing the onset of the malady to mental phenomena and not to obstructions of the spleen or viscera, Sydenham was moving towards a psychosomatic theory of hypochondriasis, one that was to be debated in the next century in England, Holland, and France.[6] Sydenham's influence on the physicians of the eighteenth century was profound: Cheyne in England, Boerhaave in Holland, La Mettrie in France. Once the theory of the nervous origins of hypochondria gained ground—here I merely note coincidence, not historical cause and effect—the disease became increasingly fashionable in England, particularly among the polite, the aristocratic, and the refined. Students of the drama will recall Scrub's denial in *The Beaux' Stratagem* (1707) of the possibility that Archer has the spleen and Mrs. Sullen's interjection, "I thought that distemper had been only proper to people of quality."

Toward the middle of the eighteenth century, hypochondria was so prevalent in people's minds and mouths that it soon assumed the abbreviated name "the hyp." Entire poems like William Somervile's *The Hyp: a Burlesque Poem in Five Canto's* (1731) and Tim Scrubb's *A Rod for the Hyp-Doctor* (1731) were devoted to this strain; others, like Malcom Flemyng's epic poem, *Neuropathia: sive de morbis hypochondriacis et hystericis, libri tres, poema medicum* (1740), were more technical and scientific. Professor Donald Davie has written that he has often "heard old fashioned and provincial persons [in England and Scotland] even in [my] own lifetime say, 'Oh, you give me the hyp,' where we should say 'You give me a pain in the neck'"[7]; and I myself have heard the expression, "You give me the pip," where "pip" may be a corruption of "hyp." As used in the early eighteenth century, the term "hyp" was perhaps not far from what our century has learned to call *Angst*. It was also used as a synonym for "lunacy," as the anonymous author of *Anti-Siris* (1744), one of the tracts in the tar-water controversy, informs us that "Berkeley tells his Countrymen, they are all mad, or *Hypochondriac*, which is but a fashionable name for Madness." Bernard Mandeville, the Dutch physician and author of *The Fable of the Bees*, seems to have understood perfectly well that hypochondriasis is a condition encompassing any number of diseases and not a specific and readily definable ailment; a condition, moreover, that hovers precariously and bafflingly in limbo between mind and body, and he stressed this as the theme of his *Treatise of the Hypochondriack and Hysteric*

Passions, Vulgarly Call'd the Hypo in Men and Vapours in Women (1711). The mental causes are noted as well in an anonymous pamphlet in the British Museum, *A Treatise on the Dismal Effects of Low-Spiritedness* (1750) and are echoed in many similar early and mid-eighteenth century works. Some medical writers of the age, like Nicholas Robinson, had reservations about the external mental bases of the hyp and preferred to discuss the condition in terms of internal physiological causes:

>...of that Disorder we call the Vapours, or *Hypochondria*; for they have no material distinctive Characters, but what arise from the same Disease affecting different Sexes, and the Vapours in Women are term'd the *Hypochondria* in Men, and they proceed from the Contraction of the Vessels being depress'd a little beneath the Balance of Nature, and the Relaxation of the Nerves at the same Time, which creates that Uneasiness and Melancholy that naturally attends Vapours, and which generally is an Intemperature of the whole Body, proceeding from a Depression of the Solids beneath the Balance of Nature; but the Intemperature of the Parts is that Peculiar Disposition whereby they favour any Disease.[8]

But the majority of medical thinkers had been persuaded that the condition was psychosomatic, and this belief was supported by research on nerves by important physicians in the 1740's and 1750's: the Monro brothers in London, Robert Whytt in Edinburgh, Albrecht von Haller in Leipzig. By mid century the condition known as the hyp was believed to be a real, not an imaginary ailment, common, peculiar in its manifestations, and indefinable, almost impossible to cure, producing very real symptoms of physical illness, and said to originate sometimes in depression and idleness. It was summed up by Robert James in his *Medicinal Dictionary* (London, 1743-45):

>If we thoroughly consider its Nature, it will be found to be a spasmodico-flatulent Disorder of the *Primae Viae*, that is, of the Stomach and Intestines, arising from an Inversion or Perversion of their peristaltic Motion, and, by the mutual consent of the Parts, throwing the whole nervous System into irregular Motions, and disturbing the whole Oeconomy of the Functions.... no part or Function of the Body escapes

the Influence of this tedious and long protracted Disease, whose Symptoms are so violent and numerous, that it is no easy Task either to enumerate or account for them.... No disease is more troublesome, either to the Patient or Physician, than hypochondriac Disorders; and it often happens, that, thro' the Fault of both, the Cure is either unnecessarily protracted, or totally frustrated; for the Patients are so delighted, not only with a Variety of Medicines, but also of Physicians.... On the contrary, few physicians are sufficiently acquainted with the true Genius and Nature of this perplexing Disorder; for which Reason they boldly prescribe almost everything contained in the Shops, not without an irreparable Injury to the Patient (article on "Hypochondriacus Morbis").

This is a more technical description than Hill gives anywhere in his handbook, but it serves well to summarize the background of the condition about which Sir John wrote.

Hill's *Hypochondriasis* adds little that is new to the theory of the disease. It incorporates much of the thinking set forth by the writings mentioned above, particularly those of George Cheyne, whose medical works *The English Malady* (1733) and *The Natural Method of Cureing the Diseases of the Body, and the Disorders of the Mind Depending on the Body* (1742) Hill knew. He is also conversant with some Continental writers on the subject, two of whom—Isaac Biberg, author of The *Oeconomy of Nature* (1751), and René Réaumur who had written a history of insects (1722)[9]—he mentions explicitly, and with William Stukeley's *Of the Spleen* (1723). Internal evidence indicates that Hill had read or was familiar with the ideas propounded in Richard Blackmore's *Treatise of the Spleen and Vapours* (1725) and Nicholas Robinson's *A New System of the Spleen, Vapours, and Hypochondriack Melancholy* (1729).

Hill's arrangement of sections is logical: he first defines the condition (I), then proceeds to discuss persons most susceptible to it (II), its major symptoms (III), consequences (IV), causes (V), and cures (VI-VIII). In the first four sections almost every statement is commonplace and requires no commentary (for example, Hill's opening remark: "To call the Hypochondriasis a fanciful malady, is ignorant and cruel. It is a real, and a sad disease: an obstruction of the spleen by thickened and distempered blood; extending itself often to the liver, and other parts; and unhappily is in England very frequent: physick scarce knows one more fertile in ill; or more difficult of cure.") His belief that the condition afflicts sedentary persons, particularly students, philosophers, theologians, and that it is not restricted to women alone—as some contemporary thinkers still maintained—is also impossible to trace to a single source, as is his description (p. 12) of the most prevalent physiological *symptoms* ("lowness of spirits, and inaptitude to motion; a disrelish of amusements, a love of solitude.... Wild thoughts; a sense of fullness") and *causes* (the poor and damp English climate and the resultant clotting of blood in the spleen) of the illness.

Sections V-VIII, dealing with causes and cures, are less commonplace and display some of Hill's eccentricities as a writer and thinker. He uses the section entitled "Cures" as a means to peddle his newly discovered cure-all, water dock,[10] which Smollett satirized through the mouth of Tabitha Bramble in *Humphry Clinker* (1771). Hill also rebelled against contemporary apothecaries and physicians who prescribed popular medicines—such as Berkeley's tar-water, Dover's mercury powders, and James's fever-powders—as universal panaceas for the cure of the hyp. "No acrid medicine must be directed, for that may act too hastily, dissolve the impacted matter at once, and let it loose, to the destruction of the sufferer; no antimonial, no mercurial, no martial preparation must be taken; in short, no chymistry: nature is the shop that heaven has set before us, and we must seek our medicine there" (p. 24). However scientifically correct Hill may have been in minimizing the efficacy of current pills and potions advertised as remedies for the hyp, he was unusual for his time in objecting so strongly to them. Less eccentric was his allegiance to the "Ancients" rather than to the "Moderns" so far as chemical treatment (i.e., restoration of the humours by chemical rearrangement) of hypochondriasis is concerned.[11] "The venerable ancients," Hill writes, "who knew not this new art, will lead us in the search; and (faithful relators as they are of truth) will tell us whence we may deduce our hope; and what we are to fear" (p. 24).

Still more idiosyncratic, perhaps, is Hill's contention (p. 25) that the air of dry, high grounds worsens the condition of the patient. Virtually every writer I have read on the subject believed that onset of the hyp was caused by one of the six non-naturals—air, diet, lack of sufficient sleep, too little or too much exercise, defective evacuation, the passions of the mind; and although some medical writers emphasized the last of these,[12] few would have concurred with Hill that the fetid air of London was less harmful than the clearer air at Highgate. All readers of the novel of the period will recall the hypochondriacal Matt Bramble's tirade against the stench of London air. Beliefs of the variety here mentioned cause me to question Hill's importance in the history of medicine; there can be no question about his contributions to the advancement of the science of botany through popularization of Linnaeus' system of bisexual classification, but Hill's medical importance is summarized best as that of a compiler. His recommendation of the study of botany as a cure for melancholics is sensible but verges on becoming "a digression in praise of the author," a poetic *apologia pro vita sua* in Augustan fashion:

For me, I should advise above all other things the study of nature. Let him begin with plants: he will here find a continual pleasure, and continual change; fertile of a thousand useful things; even of the utility we are seeking here. This will induce him to walk; and every hedge and hillock, every foot-path side, and thicket, will afford him some new object. He will be tempted to be continually in the air; and continually to change the nature and quality of the air, by visiting in succession the high lands and the low, the lawn, the heath, the forest. He will never want inducement to be abroad; and the unceasing variety of the subjects of his observation, will prevent his walking hastily: he will pursue his studies in the air; and that contemplative turn of mind, which in his closet threatened his destruction, will thus become the great means of his recovery (pp. 26-27).

Hill was forever extolling the claims of a life devoted to the study of nature, as we see in a late work, *The Virtues of British Herbs* (1770). Judicious as is the logic of this recommendation, one cannot help but feel that the emphasis here is less on diversion as a cure and more on the botanic attractions of "every hedge and hillock, every foot-path side, and thicket."

While Hill's rules and regulations regarding proper diet (Section VII) are standard, several taken almost *verbatim et literatim* from Cheyne's list in *The English Malady* (1733), his recommendation (Section VIII) of "Spleen-Wort" as the best medicine for the hypochondriac patient is not. Since Hill devotes so much space to the virtues of this herb and concludes his work extolling this plant, a word should be said about it. Throughout his life he was an active botanist. Apothecary, physician, and writer though he was, it was ultimately botany that was his ruling passion, as is made abundantly clear in his correspondence.[13] Wherever he lived—whether in the small house in St. James's Street or in the larger one on the Bayswater Road—he cultivated an herb garden that flattered his knowledge and ability. Connoisseurs raved about its species and considered it one of the showpieces of London. His arrogant personality alone prevented him from becoming the first Keeper of the Apothecary's Garden in Chelsea, although he was for a time superintendent to the Dowager Princess of Wales's gardens at Kensington Palace and at Kew. His interest in cultivation of herbs nevertheless continued; over the years Hill produced more than thirty botanical works, many of them devoted to the medical virtues of rare herbs such as "Spleen-Wort." Among these are *The British Herbal* (1756), *On the Virtues of Sage in Lengthening Human Life* (1763), *Centaury, the Great Stomachic* (1765), *Polypody* (1768), *A Method of Curing Jaundice* (1768), *Instances of the Virtue of Petasite Root* (1771), and *Twenty Five New Plants* (1773).[14] It is therefore not surprising that he should believe a specific herb to be the best remedy for a complicated medical condition. Nor is his reference to the Ancients as authority for the herbal pacification of an inflamed spleen surprising in the light of his researches: he was convinced that every illness could be cured by taking an appropriate herb or combination of herbs. Whereas a few nonmedical writers—such as John Wesley in *Primitive Physick* (1747)—had advocated the taking of one or two herbs in moderate dosage as anti-hysterics (the eighteenth-century term for all cures of the hyp), no medical writer of the century ever promoted the use of herbs to the extent that Hill did. In fairness to him, it is important to note that his herbal remedies were harmless and that many found their way into the official *London Pharmacopeia*. "The virtues of this smooth Spleen-wort," he insists, "have stood the test of ages; and the plant every where retained its name and credit: and one of our good herbarists, who had seen a wonderful case of a swoln spleen, so big, and hard as to be felt with terror, brought back to a state of nature by it" (p. 37).[15] The greatest portion of Hill's concluding section combines advertisement for the powder medicine he was himself manufacturing at a handsome profit together with a protest against competing apothecaries: "An intelligent person was directed to go to the medicinal herb shops in the several markets, and buy some of this Spleen-wort; the name was written, and shewn to every one; every shop received his money, and almost every one sold a different plant, under the name of this: but what is very striking, not one of them the right" (p. 42).

Treatises on hypochondriasis did not cease to be printed after Hill's in 1766, but continued to issue from the presses into the nineteenth century. A good example of this is the tome by John Reid, physician to the Finsbury Dispensary in London, *Essays on Insanity, Hypochondriasis and Other Nervous Affections* (1816), which summarizes theories of the malady.[16] A bibliographical study of such works would probably reveal a larger number of titles in the nineteenth century than in the previous one, but by this time the nature and definition of hypochondria had changed significantly.

If John Hill's volume is not an important contribution in the history of medicine, it is a lucid and brief exposition of many of the best ideas that had been thought and written on the hyp, with the exception of his uninhibited prescribing of herbal medicines as cure-alls. An understanding of this disease is essential for readers of neoclassical English literature, especially when we reflect upon the fact that some of the best literature of the period was composed by writers whom it afflicted. It is perhaps not without significance that the greatest poet of the Augustan age, Alexander Pope, thought it necessary as he lay on his deathbed in May 1744 to exclaim with his last breath, "I never was hippish in my whole life."[17]

University of California,

Los Angeles

NOTES TO THE INTRODUCTION

[1] The text here reproduced is that of the copy in the Library of the Royal Society of Medicine, London. Title pages of different copies of the first edition of 1766 vary. For example, the title page of the copy in the British Museum reads, *Hypochondriasis; a Practical Treatise On the Nature and Cure of that Disorder, Commonly called the Hyp and the Hypo.* The copy in the Royal Society of Medicine contains, among other additions, the words "by Sir John Hill" in pencil, and "8vo Lond. 1766," written in ink and probably a later addition.

[2] Melancholy, hypochondriasis, and the spleen were considered in the seventeenth and eighteenth centuries to be one complex condition, a malady rather than a malaise, which is but a symptom. Distinctions among these, of interest primarily to medical historians, cannot be treated here. As good a definition as any is found in Dr. Johnson's *Dictionary* (1755): "Hypochondriacal.... 1. Melancholy; disordered in the imagination.... 2. Producing melancholy...." The literature of melancholy has been surveyed in part by C. A. Moore, "The English Malady," *Backgrounds of English Literature 1700-1760* (Minneapolis, 1953), pp. 179-235. In medical parlance, "hypochondria" means the soft parts of the body below the costal cartilages, and the singular form of the word, "hypochondrium," means the viscera situated in the hypochondria, i.e., the liver, gall bladder, and spleen.

[3] See Samuel Clifford's *The Signs and Causes of Melancholy, with directions suited to the case of those who are afflicted with it. Collected out of the works of Mr. Richard Baxter* (London, 1716) in the British Museum.

[4] *Backgrounds of English Literature*, p. 179.

[5] See my forthcoming biography, _The Literary Quack: A Life of 'Sir' John Hill of London_, and John Kennedy's *Some Remarks on the Life and Writings of Dr. J—— H——, Inspector General of Great Britain* (London, 1752).

[6] For some of this background see L. J. Rather, *Mind and Body in Eighteenth Century Medicine: A Study Based on Jerome Gaub's De Regimine Mentis* (London, 1965), pp. 135-90 *passim*.

[7] *Science and Literature 1700-1740* (London, 1964), pp. 50-51.

[8] *A New Theory of Physick* (London, 1725), p. 56.

[9] Biberg was a Swedish naturalist and had studied botany under Linnaeus in Uppsala; Réaumur, a French botanist, had contributed papers to the *Philosophical Transactions* of the Royal Society in London.

[10] *The Power of Water-Dock against the Scurvy whether in the Plain Root or Essence....* (London, 1765), had been published six months earlier than *Hypochondriasis* and had earned Hill a handsome profit.

[11] I have treated aspects of this subject in my article, "Matt Bramble and The Sulphur Controversy in the XVIIIth Century: Medical Background of *Humphry Clinker*," *JHI*, XXVIII (1967), 577-90.

[12] See, for example, Jeremiah Waineright, *A Mechanical Account of the Non-Naturals* (1707); John Arbuthnot, *An Essay Concerning the Effects of Air on Human Bodies* (1733); Frank Nichols, *De Anima Medica* (1750).

[13] Hill's correspondence is not published but shall be printed as an appendix to my forthcoming biography.

[14] I have discussed some of these works in connection with the medical background of John Wesley's *Primitive Physick* (1747). See G. S. Rousseau, *Harvard Library Bulletin*, XVI (1968), 242-56.

[15] It is difficult to know with certainty when Hill first became interested in the herb. He mentions it in passing in *The British Herbal* (1756), I, 526 and may have sold it as early as 1742 when he opened an apothecary shop.

[16] Reid's dissertation at Edinburgh, entitled *De Insania* (1798), contains materials on the relationship of the imagination to all forms of mental disturbance. Secondary literature on hypochondria is plentiful. Works include: R. H. Gillespie, *Hypochondria* (London, 1928), William K. Richmond, *The English Disease* (London, 1958), Charles Chenevix Trench, *The Royal Malady* (New York, 1964), and Ilza Vieth, *Hysteria: The History of a Disease* (Chicago, 1965), and "On Hysterical and Hypochondriacal Afflictions," *Bulletin of the History of Medicine*, XXX (1956), 233-40.

[17] Joseph Spence, *Observations, Anecdotes, and Characters of Books and Men*, ed. James M. Osborn (Oxford, 1966), I, 264.

I am indebted to A. D. Morris, M.D., F.R.S.M., for help of various sorts in writing this introduction.

BIBLIOGRAPHICAL NOTE

The text of this facsimile of *Hypochondriasis* is reproduced from a copy in the Library of the Royal Society of Medicine, London.

SECT. I.

The Nature of the Disorder.

To call the Hypochondriasis a fanciful malady, is ignorant and cruel. It is a real, and a sad disease: an obstruction of the spleen by thickened and distempered blood; extending itself often to the liver, and other parts; and unhappily is in England very frequent: physick scarce knows one more fertile in ill; or more difficult of cure.

The blood is a mixture of many fluids, which, in a state of health, are so combined, that the whole passes freely through its appointed vessels; but if by the loss of the thinner parts, the rest becomes too gross to be thus carried through, it will stop where the circulation has least power; and having thus stopped it will accumulate; heaping by degrees obstruction on obstruction.

Health and chearfulness, and the quiet exercise of mind, depend upon a perfect circulation: is it a wonder then, when this becomes impeded the body looses of its health, and the temper of its sprightliness? to be otherwise would be the miracle; and he inhumanly insults the afflicted, who calls all this a voluntary frowardness. Its slightest state brings with it sickness, anguish and oppression; and innumerable ills follow its advancing steps, unless prevented by timely care; till life itself grows burthensome.

The disease was common in antient Greece; and her physicians understood it, better than those perhaps of later times, in any other country; who though happy in many advantages these fathers of the science could not have, yet want the great assistance of frequent watching it in all its stages.

Those venerable writers have delivered its nature, and its cure: in the first every thing now shews they were right; and what they have said as to the latter will be found equally true and certain. This, so far as present experience has confirmed it, and no farther, will be here laid before the afflicted in a few plain words.

SECT. II.

Persons Subject to it.

Fatigue of mind, and great exertion of its powers often give birth to this disease; and always tend to encrease it. The finer spirits are wasted by the labour of the brain: the Philosopher rises from his study more exhausted than the Peasant leaves his drudgery; without the benefit that he has from exercise. Greatness of mind, and steady virtue; determined resolution, and manly firmness, when put in action, and intent upon their object, all also lead to it: perhaps whatever tends to the ennobling of the soul has equal share in bringing on this weakness of the body.

From this we may learn easily who are the men most subject to it; the grave and studious, those of a sedate temper and enlarged understanding, the learned and wise, the virtuous and the valiant: those whom it were the interest of the world to wish were free from this and every other illness; and who perhaps, except for this alloy, would have too large a portion of human happiness.

Though these are most, it is not these alone, who are subject to it. There are countries where it is endemial, and in other places some have the seeds of it in their constitution; and in some it takes rise from accidents. In these last it is the easiest of cure; and in the first most difficult.

Beside the Greeks already named, the Jews of old time were heavily afflicted with this disease; and in their descendants to this day it is often constitutional: the Spaniards have it almost to a man; and so have the American Indians. Perhaps the character of these several nations may be connected with it. The steady honour, and firm valour of the Spaniard, very like that of the ancient Doric nation, who followed the flute not the trumpet to the field; and met the enemy, not with shouts and fury, but with a determined virtue: it is the temper of the Hypochondriac to be slow, but unmoveably resolved: the Jew has shewn this mistakenly, but almost miraculously; and the poor Indian, untaught as he is, faces all peril with composure, and sings his death-song with an unalter'd countenance.

Among particular persons the most inquiring and contemplative are those who suffer oftenest by this disease; and of all degrees of men I think the clergy. I do not mean the hunting, shooting, drinking clergy, who bear the tables of the great; but the retir'd and conscientious; such as attend in midnight silence to their duty; and seek in their own cool breasts, or wheresoever else they may be found, new admonitions for an age plunged in new vices. To this disease we owe the irreparable loss of Dr. Young; and the present danger of many other the best and most improved amongst us. May what is here to be proposed assist in their preservation!

The Geometrician or the learned Philosopher of whatever denomination, whose course of study fixes his eye for ever on one object, his mind intensely and continually employed upon one thought, should be warned also that he is in danger; or if he find himself already afflicted, he should be told that the same course of life, which brought it on, will, without due care, encrease it to the most dreaded violence.

The middle period of life is that in which there is the greatest danger of an attack from this disease; and the latter end of autumn, when the summer heats have a little time been over, is the season when in our climate its first assaults are most to be expected. The same time of the year always increases the disorder in those who have been before afflicted with it; and it is a truth must be confessed, that from its first attack the patient grows continually, though slowly, worse; unless a careful regimen prevent it.

The constitutions most liable to this obstruction are the lean, and dark complexioned; the grave and sedentary. Let such watch the first symptoms; and obviate, (as they may with ease) that which it will be much more difficult to remove.

It is happy a disease, wherein the patient must do a great deal for himself, falls, for the most part, upon those who have the powers of reason strongest. Let them only be aware of this, that the distemper naturally disposes them to inactivity; and reason will have no use unless accompanied with resolution to enforce it.

Though the physician can do something toward the cure, much more depends upon the patient; and here his constancy of mind will be employed most happily. No one is better qualified to judge on a fair hearing what course is the most fit; and having made that choice, he must with patience wait its good effects. Diseases that come on slowly must have time for curing; an attention to the first appearances of the disorder will be always happiest; because when least established it is easiest overthrown: but when that happy period has been neglected, he must wait the effects of such a course as will dilute and melt the obstructing matter gradually; for till that be done it is not only vain, but sometimes dangerous, to attempt its expulsion from the body.

The blood easily separates itself into the grosser and the thinner parts: we see this in bleeding; and from the toughness of the red cake may guess how very difficult it will be to dissolve a substance of like firmness in the vessels of the body. That it can thus become thickened within the body, a Pleurisy shews us too evidently: in that case it is brought on suddenly, and with inflammation; in this other, slowly and without; and here, even before it forms the obstruction, can bring on many mischiefs. Various causes can produce the same effect, but that in all cases operates most durably, which operates most slowly. The watery part of the blood is its mild part; in the remaining gross matter of it, are acrid salts and burning oils, and these, when destitute of that happy dilution nature gives them in a healthy body, are capable of doing great mischief to the tender vessels in which they are kept stagnant.

SECT. III.

The Symptoms of the Disorder.

The first and lightest of the signs that shew this illness are a lowness of spirits, and inaptitude to motion; a disrelish of amusements, a love of solitude and a habit of thinking, even on trifling subjects, with too much steadiness. A very little help may combat these: but if that indolence which is indeed a part of the disorder, will neglect them; worse must be expected soon to follow.

Wild thoughts; a sense of fullness, weight, and oppression in the body, a want of appetite, or, what is worse, an appetite without digestion; for these are the conditions of different states of the disease, a fullness and a difficulty of breathing after meals, a straitness of the breast, pains and flatulencies in the bowels, and an unaptness to discharge their contents.

The pulse becomes low, weak, and unequal; and there are frequent palpitations of the heart, a little dark-coloured urine is voided at some times; and a flood of colourless and insipid at others; relieving for a moment, but increasing the distemper: there is in some cases also a continual teazing cough, with a choaking stoppage in the throat at times; then heartburn, sickness, hardness of the belly, and a costive habit, or a tormenting and vain irritation.

The lips turn pale, the eyes loose their brightness and by degrees the white grows as it were greenish, the gums want their due firmness, with their proper colour; and an unpleasing foulness grows upon the teeth: the inside of the mouth is pale and furred, and the throat dry and husky: the colour of the skin is pale (though there are periods when the face is florid) and as the obstruction gathers ground, and more affects the liver, the whole body becomes yellow, tawny, greenish, and at length of that deep and dusky hue, to which men of swift imagination have given the name of blackness.

These symptoms do not all appear in any one period of the disease, or in one case, but at one time or other all of them, as well as those which follow: the flesh becomes cold to the touch, though the patient does not himself perceive it; the limbs grow numbed and torpid, the breathing dull and slow, and the voice hollow; and usually the appetite in this period declines, and comes almost to nothing: night sweats come on, black swellings appear on the veins, the flesh wastes and the breast becomes flat and hollow: the mouth is full of a thin spittle, the head is dizzy and confus'd, and sometimes there is an unconquerable numbness in the organs of speech.

I have known the temporary silence that follows upon this last symptom become a jest to the common herd; and the unhappy patient, instead of compassion and assistance, receive the reproof of sullenness, from those who should have known and acted better.

About twenty years ago I met on a visit at Catthorpe in Leicestershire a young gentleman of distinguished learning and abilities, who at certain times was speechless. The vulgar thought it a pretence: and a jocose lady, where he was at tea with company, putting him as she said to a trial, poured out a dish very strong and without sugar. He drank it and returned the cup with a bow of great reserve, and his eye bent on the ground: she then filled the cup with sugar, and pouring weak tea on it, sent it him: he drank that too, looked at her steadily, and blushed for her. The lady declared the man was dumb; the rest thought him perverse, and obstinate; but a constant and steady perseverance in an easy method cured him.

All these are miseries which the disease, while it retains its natural form, can bring upon the patient; and thus he will in time be worn out, and led miserably, though slowly, to the grave. Let him not indulge his inactivity so far as to give way to this, because it is represented as far off; the disease may suddenly and frightfully change its nature; and swifter evils follow.

SECT. IV.

The Danger.

We have done with the obstruction considered in itself; but this, though often unsurmountable by art, at least by the methods now in use, will be sometimes broken through at once by nature, or by accidents; and bring on fatal evils. These are strictly different diseases, and are no otherway concerned here, than as the consequences of that of which we are treating.

The thick and glutinous blood which has so long stagnated in the spleen, will have in that time altered its nature, and acquired a very great degree of acrimony: while it lies dormant, this does no more mischiefs, than those named already; but when violent exercise, a fit of outrageous anger, or any thing else that suddenly shocks and disturbs the frame, puts it in motion, it melts at once into a kind of liquid putrefaction. Being now thin, it mixes itself readily with the blood again, and brings on putrid fevers; destroys the substance of the spleen itself, or being thrown upon some other of the viscera, corrodes them, and leads on this way a swift and miserable death. If it fall upon the liver, its tender pulpy substance is soon destroyed, jaundices beyond the help of art first follow, then dropsies and all their train of misery; if on lungs, consumptions; if on the brain, convulsions, epilepsy, palsy, apoplexy; if on the surface, leprosy.

The intention of cure is to melt this coagulation softly, not to break it violently; and then to give it a very gentle passage through the bowels. There is no safe way for it to take but that; and even that when urged too far may bring on fatal dysenteries.

Let none wonder at the sudden devastation which sometimes arises from this long stagnant matter, when liquified too hastily: how long, how many years the impacted matter will continue quiet in a schirrous tumour of the breast; but being once put in motion, whether from accident, or in the course of nature, what can describe; or what can stop its havock!

Instances of the other are too frequent. A nobleman the other day died paralytick: dissection shewed a spleen consumed by an abscess, formed from the dissolved matter of such an obstruction: and 'tis scarce longer since, a learned gentleman, who had been several years lost to his friends, by the extreams of a Hypochondriacal disorder, seem'd gradually without assistance to recover: but the lungs suffered while the spleen was freed; and he died very soon of what is called a galloping consumption.

When the obstruction is great and of long continuance, if it be thus hastily moved, the consequence is, equally, a sudden and a miserable death, whether, like the matter of a cancer, it remains in its place; or like that of a bad small pox, be thrown upon some other vital part.

Let not the patient be too much alarmed; this is laid down to caution, not to terrify him: it is fit he should know his danger, and attend to it; for the prevention is easy; and the cure, even of the most advanced stages, when undertaken by gentle means, is not at all impracticable: to assist the physician, let him look into himself, and recollect the source of his complaint. This he may judge of from the following notices.

SECT. V.

The Causes of the Hypochondriasis.

The obstruction which forms this disease, may take its origin from different accidents: a fever ill cured has often caused it; or the piles, which had been used to discharge largely, ceasing; a marshy soil, poisoned with stagnant water, has given it to some persons; and altho' indolence and inactivity are oftenest at the root, yet it has arisen from too great exercise.

Real grief has often brought it on; and even love, for sometimes that is real. Study and fixed attention of the mind have been accused before; and add to these the stooping posture of the body, which most men use, though none should use it, in writing and in reading. This has contributed too much to it; but of all other things night studies are the most destructive. The steady stillness, and dusky habit of all nature in those hours, enforce, encourage, and support that settled gloom, which rises from fixt thought; and sinks the body to the grave; even while it carries up the mind to heaven. He who would have his lamp

At midnight hour
Be seen in some high lonely tower,[18]   will   waste   the   flame   of   this unheeded life: and while he labours to unsphere the spirit of Plato[18] will let loose his own.

SECT. V.

The Cure of the Hypochondriasis.

Let him who would escape the mischiefs of an obstructed spleen, avoid the things here named: and let him who suffers from the malady, endeavour to remember to which of them it has been owing; for half the hope depends upon that knowledge.

Nature has sometimes made a cure herself, and we should watch her ways; for art never is so right as when it imitates her: sometimes the patient's own resolution has set him free. This is always in his power, and at all times will do wonders.

The bleeding of the piles, from nature's single efforts, has at once cured a miserable man; where their cessation was the cause of the disorder. A leprosy has appeared upon the skin, and all the symptoms of the former sickness vanished. This among the Jews happened often: both diseases we know were common among them: and I have here seen something very like it: Water-Dock has thrown out scorbutic eruptions, and all the former symptoms of an Hypochondriacal disorder have disappeared: returning indeed when these were unadvisedly struck in; but keeping off entirely when they were better treated. A natural purging unsuppressed has sometimes done the same good office: but this is hazardous.

It is easy to be directed from such instances; only let us take the whole along with us. Bleeding would have answered nature's purpose, if she could not have opened of herself the hæmorrhoidal vessels; but he who should give medicines for that purpose, might destroy his patient by too great disturbance. If a natural looseness may perform the cure, so may an artificial; when the original source of the disorder points that way. But these are helps that take place only in particular cases.

The general and universal method of cure must be by some mild and gently resolving medicine, under the influence of which the obstructing matter may be voided that, or some other way with safety. The best season to undertake this is the autumn, but even here there must be caution.

In the first place, no strong evacuating remedy must be given; for that, by carrying off the thinner parts of the juices, will tend to thicken the remainder; and certainly encrease the distemper. No acrid medicine must be directed, for that may act too hastily, dissolve the impacted matter at once, and let it loose, to the destruction of the sufferer; no antimonial, no mercurial, no martial preparation must be taken; in short, no chymistry: nature is the shop that heaven has set before us, and we must seek our medicine there. The venerable ancients, who knew not this new art, will lead us in the search; and (faithful relators as they are of truth) will tell us whence we may deduce our hope; and what we are to fear.

But prior to the course of any medicine, and as an essential to any good hope from it, the patient must prescribe himself a proper course of life, and a well chosen diet: let us assist him in his choice; and speak of this first, as it comes first in order.

SECT. VI.

Rules of Life for Hypochondriac Persons.

Air and exercise, as they are the best preservers of health, and greatest assistants in the cure of all long continued diseases, will have their full effect in this; but there requires some caution in the choice, and management of them. It is common to think the air of high grounds best; but experience near home shews otherwise: the Hypochondriac patient is always worse at Highgate even than in London.

The air he breathes should be temperate; not exposed to the utmost violences of heat and cold, and the swift changes from one to the other; which are most felt on those high grounds. The side of a hill is the best place for him: and though wet grounds are hurtful; yet let there be the shade of trees, to tempt him often to a walk; and soften by their exhalation the over dryness of the air.

The exercise he takes should be frequent; but not violent. Motion preserves the firmness of the parts, and elasticity of the vessels; it prevents that aggregation of thick humours which he is most to fear. A sedentary life always produces weakness, and that mischief always follows: weak eyes are gummy, weak lungs are clogged with phlegm, and weak bowels waste themselves in vapid diarrhœas.

Let him invite himself abroad, and let his friends invite him by every innocent inducement. For me, I should advise above all other things the study of nature. Let him begin with plants: he will here find a continual pleasure, and continual change; fertile of a thousand useful things; even of the utility we are seeking here. This will induce him to walk; and every hedge and hillock, every foot-path side, and thicket, will afford him some new object. He will be tempted to be continually in the air, and continually to change the nature and quality of the air, by visiting in succession the high lands and the low, the lawn, the heath, the forest. He will never want inducement to be abroad; and the unceasing variety of the subjects of his observation, will prevent his walking hastily: he will pursue his studies in the air; and that contemplative turn of mind, which in his closet threatened his destruction, will thus become the great means of his recovery.

If the mind tire upon this, from the repeated use, another of nature's kingdoms opens itself at once upon him; the plant he is weary of observing, feeds some insect he may examine; nor is there a stone that lies before his foot, but may afford instruction and amusement.

Even what the vulgar call the most abject things will shew a wonderful utility; and lead the mind, in pious contemplation higher than the stars. The poorest moss that is trampled under foot, has its important uses: is it at the bottom of a wood we find it? why there it shelters the fallen seeds; hides them from birds, and covers them from frost; and thus becomes the foster father of another forest! creeps it along the surface of a rock? even there its good is infinite! its small roots run into the stone, and the rains make their way after them; the moss having lived its time dies; it rots and with the mouldered fragments of the stone forms earth; wherein, after a few successions, useful plants may grow, and feed more useful cattle![19]

Is there a weed more humble in its aspect, more trampled on, or more despised than knot grass! no art can get the better of its growth, no labour can destroy it; 'twere pity if they could, for the thing lives where nothing would of use to us; and its large and most wonderfully abundant seeds, feed in hard winters, half the birds of Heaven.

What the weak moss performs upon the rock the loathed toadstool brings about in timber: is an oak dead where man's eye will not find it? this fungus roots itself upon the bark, and rots the wood beneath it; hither the beetle creeps for shelter, and for sustenance; him the woodpecker follows as his prey; and while he tears the tree in search of him, he scatters it about the ground; which it manures.

Nor is it the beetle alone that thus insinuates itself into the substance of the vegetable tribe: the tender aphide[20], whom a touch destroys, burrows between the two skins of a leaf, for shelter from his winged enemies; tracing, with more than Dedalæan art, his various meanders; and veining the green surface with these white lines more beautifully than the best Ægyptian marble.

'Twere endless to proceed; nor is it needful: one object will not fail to lead on to another, and every where the goodness of his God will shine before him even in what are thought the vilest things; his greatness in the lead of them.

Let him pursue these thoughts, and seek abroad the objects and the instigations to them: but let him in these and all other excursions avoid equally the dews of early morning, and of evening.

The more than usual exercise of this prescription will dispose him to more than customary sleep, let him indulge it freely; so far from hurting, it will help his cure.

Let him avoid all excesses: drink need scarce be named, for we are writing to men of better and of nobler minds, than can be tempted to that humiliating vice. Those who in this disorder have too great an appetite, must not indulge it; much eaten was never well digested: but of all excesses the most fatal in this case is that of venery. It is the excess we speak of.

SECT. VII.

The proper Diet.

In the first place acids must be avoided carefully; and all things that are in a state of fermentation, for they will breed acidity. Provisions hardened by salting never should be tasted; much less those cured by smoking, and by salting. Bacon is indigestible in an Hypochondriac stomach; and hams, impregnated as is now the custom, with acid fumes from the wood fires over which they are hung, have that additional mischief.

Milk ought to be a great article in the diet: and even in this there should be choice. The milk of grass-fed cows has its true quality: no other. There are a multitude of ways in which this may be made a part both of our foods and drinks, and they should all be used.

The great and general caution is that the diet be at all times of a kind loosening and gently stimulating; light but not acrid. Veal, lamb, fowls, lobsters, crabs, craw-fish, fresh water fish and mutton broth, with plenty of boiled vegetables, are always right; and give enough variety.

Raw vegetables are all bad: sour wines, old cheese, and bottled beer are things never to be once tasted. Indeed much wine is wrong, be it of what kind soever. It is the first of cordials; and as such I would have it taken in this disease when it is wanted: plainly as a medicine, rather than a part of diet. Malt liquor carefully chosen is certainly the best drink. This must be neither new, nor tending to sourness; perfectly clear, and of a moderate strength: it is the native liquor of our country, and the most healthful.

Too much tea weakens; and even sugar is in this disorder hurtful: but honey may supply its place in most things; and this is not only harmless but medicinal; a very powerful dissolvent of impacted humours, and a great deobstruent.

What wine is drank should be of some of the sweet kinds. Old Hock has been found on enquiry to yield more than ten times the acid of the sweet wines; and in red Port, at least in what we are content to call so, there is an astringent quality, that is most mischievous in these cases: it is said there is often alum in it: how pregnant with mischief that must be to persons whose bowels require to be kept open, is most evident. Summer fruits perfectly ripe are not only harmless but medicinal; but if eaten unripe they will be very prejudicial. A light supper, which will leave an appetite for a milk breakfast, is always right; this will not let the stomach be ravenous for dinner, as it is apt to be in those who make that their only meal.

One caution more must be given, and it may seem a strange one: it is that the patient attend regularly to his hours of eating. We have to do with men for the most part whose soul is the great object of their regard; but let them not forget they have a body.

The late Dr. Stukely has told me, that one day by appointment visiting Sir Isaac Newton, the servant told him, he was in his study. No one was permitted to disturb him there; but as it was near dinner time, the visitor sat down to wait for him. After a time dinner was brought in; a boil'd chicken under a cover. An hour pass'd, and Sir Isaac did not appear. The doctor eat the fowl, and covering up the empty dish, bad them dress their master another. Before that was ready, the great man came down; he apologiz'd for his delay, and added, "give me but leave to take my short dinner, and I shall be at your service; I am fatigued and faint." Saying this, he lifted up the cover; and without any emotion, turned about to Stukely with a smile; "See says he, what we studious people are, I forgot I had din'd."

SECT. VIII.

The Medicine.

'Tis the ill fate of this disease, more than of all others to be misunderstood at first, and thence neglected; till the physician shakes his head at a few first questions. None steals so fatally upon the sufferer: its advances are by very slow degrees; but every day it grows more difficult of cure.

That this obstruction in the spleen is the true malady, the cases related by the antients, present observation, and the unerring testimonies of dissections leave no room to doubt. Being understood, the path is open where to seek a remedy: and our best guides in this, as in the former instance, will be those venerable Greeks; who saw a thousand of these cases, where we see one; and with less than half our theory, cured twice as many patients.

One established doctrine holds place in all these writers; that whatever by a hasty fermentation dissolves the impacted matter of the obstruction, and sends it in that state into the blood, does incredible mischief: but that whatever medicine softens it by slow degrees, and, as it melts, delivers it to the bowels without disturbance; will cure with equal certainty and safety.

For this good purpose, they knew and tried a multitude of herbs; but in the end they fixed on one: and on their repeated trials of this, they banished all the rest. This stood alone for the cure of the disease; and from its virtue received the name of Spleen-wort[21]. O wise and happy Greeks! authors of knowledge and perpetuators of it! With them the very name they gave a plant declared its virtues: with us, a writer calls a plant from some friend; that the good gardener who receives the honour, may call another by his name who gave it. We now add the term *smooth* to this herb, to distinguish it from another, called by the same general term, though not much resembling it.

The virtues of this smooth Spleen-wort have flood the test of ages; and the plant every where retained its name and credit: and one of our good herbalists, who had seen a wonderful case of a swoln spleen, so big, and hard as to be felt with terror, brought back to a state of nature by it; and all the miserable symptoms vanish; thought Spleen-wort not enough expressive of its excellence; but stamp'd on it the name of Milt-waste.

In the Greek Islands now, the use of it is known to every one; and even the lazy monks who take it, are no longer splenetic. In the west of England, the rocks are stripped of it with diligence; and every old woman tells you how charming that leaf is for bookish men: in Russia they use a plant of this kind in their malt liquor: it came into fashion there for the cure of this disease; which from its constant use is scarce known any longer; and they suppose 'tis added to their liquor for a flavour.

The antients held it in a kind of veneration; and used what has been called a superstition in the gathering it. It was to be taken up with a sharp knife, without violence, and laid upon the clean linen: no time but the still darkness of the night was proper, and even the moon was not to shine upon it[22]. I know they have been ridiculed for this; for nothing is so vain as learned ignorance: but let me be permitted once to vindicate them.

The plant has leaves that can close in their sides; and their under part is covered thick with a yellow powder, consisting of the seeds, and seed vessels: in these they knew the virtue most resided: this was the golden dust[23] they held so valuable; and this they knew they could not be too cautious to preserve. They were not ignorant of the sleep of plants; a matter lately spoken of by some, as if a new discovery; and being sensible that light, a dry air, an expanded leaf, and a tempestuous season, were the means of losing this fine dust; and knowing also that darkness alone brought on that closing of the leaf which thence has been called sleep; and which helped to defend and to secure it, they therefore took such time, and used such means as could best preserve the plant entire; and even save what might be scattered from it.—And now where is their superstition?

From this plant thus collected they prepared a medicine, which in a course of forty days scarce ever failed to make a perfect cure.

We have the plant wild with us; and till the fashion of rough chemical preparations took off our attention from these gentler remedies, it was in frequent use and great repute. I trust it will be so again: and many thank me for restoring it to notice.

Spleen-wort gives out its virtues freely in a tincture; and a small dose of this, mixing readily with the blood and juices, gradually dissolves the obstruction; and by a little at a time delivers its contents to be thrown off without pain, from the bowels. Let this be done while the viscera are yet sound and the cure is perfect. More than the forty days of the Greek method is scarce ever required; much oftener two thirds of that time suffice; and every day, from the first dose of it, the patient feels the happy change that is growing in his constitution. His food no more turns putrid on his stomach, but yields its healthful nourishment. The swelling after meals therefore vanishes; and with that goes the lowness, and anxiety, the difficult breath, and the distracting cholick: he can bear the approach of rainy weather without pain; he finds himself more apt for motion, and ready to take that exercise which is to be assistant in his cure; life seems no longer burthensome. His bowels get into the natural condition of health, and perform their office once at least a day; better if a little more: the dull and dead colour of his skin goes off, his lips grow red again, and every sign of health returns.

Let him who takes the medicine, say whether any thing here be exaggerated. Let him, if he pleases to give himself the trouble, talk over with me, or write to me, this gradual decrease of his complaints, as he proceeds in his cure. My uncertain state of health does not permit me to practise physic in the usual way, but I am very desirous to do what good I can, and shall never refuse my advice, such as it may be, to any person rich or poor, in whatever manner he may apply for it. I shall refer him to no apothecary, whose bills require he should be drenched with potions; but tell him, in this as in all other cases, where to find some simple herb; which he may if he please prepare himself; or if he had rather spare that trouble, may have it so prepared from me.

With regard to Spleen-wort, no method of using it is more effectual than simply taking it in powder; the only advantage of a tincture, is that a proper dose may be given, and yet the stomach not be loaded with so large a quantity: it is an easier and pleasanter method, and nothing more.

If any person choose to take it in the other way, I should still wish him once at least to apply to me; that he may be assured what he is about to take is the right plant. Abuses in medicines are at this time very great, and in no instance worse than what relates to herbs. The best of our physicians have complained upon this head with warmth, but without redress: they know the virtues and the value of many of our native plants, but dread to prescribe them; lest some wrong thing should be administered in their place; perhaps inefficacious, perhaps mischievous, nay it may be fatal. The few simple things I direct are always before me; and it will at all times be a pleasure to me, in this and any other instance, to see whether what any person is about to take be right. I have great obligations to the public, and this is the best return that I know how to make.

To see the need of such a caution, hear a transaction but of yesterday! An intelligent person was directed to go to the medicinal herb shops in the several markets, and buy some of this Spleen-wort; the name was written, and shewn to every one; every shop received his money, and almost every one sold a different plant, under the name of this: but what is very striking, not one of them the right. Such is the chance of health in those hands through which the best means of it usually pass; even in the most regular course of application.

I would not be understood to limit the little services I may this way be able to render the afflicted, to this single instance; much less to propose to myself any advantages from it. Whoever pleases will be welcome to me, upon any such occasion; and whatever be the herb on which he places a dependance, he shall be shewn it growing. I once recommended a garden to be established for this use, at the public expence: one great person has put it in my power to answer all its purposes.

FINIS.

Footnotes:

[18] Milton's Penseroso.
[19] Biberg.
[20] Reaumur.
[21] ασπλενον
[22] Silente Luna.
[23] Pulvis Aureus.

www.ingramcontent.com/pod-product-compliance
Lightning Source LLC
Chambersburg PA
CBHW050029230526
45470CB00003B/1188

JOSEPH GARCIA
Foreword by Connie Book, President, Elon University

WHEN *the* CAP FALLS

Ten Principles for a College Graduate to Launch a Career

outskirts press

When the Cap Falls
Ten Principles for a College Graduate to Launch a Career
All Rights Reserved.
Copyright © 2019 Joseph Garcia
v2.0

The opinions expressed in this manuscript are solely the opinions of the author and do not represent the opinions or thoughts of the publisher. The author has represented and warranted full ownership and/or legal right to publish all the materials in this book.

This book may not be reproduced, transmitted, or stored in whole or in part by any means, including graphic, electronic, or mechanical without the express written consent of the publisher except in the case of brief quotations embodied in critical articles and reviews.

Outskirts Press, Inc.
http://www.outskirtspress.com

ISBN: 978-1-9772-0921-4

Cover Photo © 2019 www.gettyimages.com. All rights reserved - used with permission.

Outskirts Press and the "OP" logo are trademarks belonging to Outskirts Press, Inc.

PRINTED IN THE UNITED STATES OF AMERICA